LOW POTASSIUM FOOD LISTS

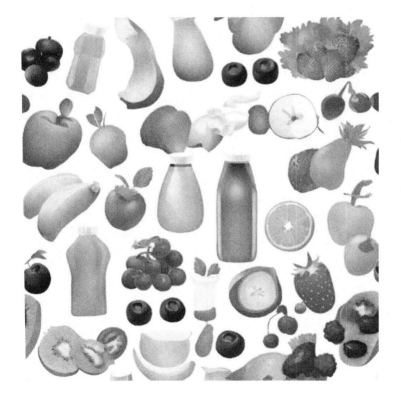

LYSANDRA QUINN

TABLE OF CONTENTS

INTRODUCTION...1

CHAPTER 1 5

What is Potassium?...5

  Why is Low Potassium Important?.................................... 6

  Who Should Follow a Low Potassium Diet?........................... 7

CHAPTER 2 9

LOW-POTASSIUM FOOD CATEGORIES 9

  Low-Potassium Fruits 9

  Low-Potassium Vegetables... 15

  Low-Potassium Protein.. 20

  Low-Potassium Dairy and Alternatives.............................. 25

  Low-Potassium Grains and Cereals 30

  Low-Potassium Snacks and Sweets 35

CONCLUSION 41

BONUS: 43

10 LOW-POTASSIUM RECIPES 43

  Grilled Chicken Breast with Lemon and Herbs...................... 43

  Baked Salmon with Dill... 45

Quinoa and Black Bean Salad.. 47

Vegetable Stir-Fry.. 49

Turkey and Vegetable Soup.. 51

Egg White Omelets with Spinach and Tomatoes 53

Low-Potassium Fruit Salad... 55

Low-Potassium Avocado and Tomato Salsa 57

Low-Potassium Tuna Salad 59

Low-Potassium Baked Sweet Potatoes..................................... 61

INTRODUCTION

In the quiet corners of my life, I stumbled upon a secret; a secret that would alter the course of my career and ignite my passion for creating a lifeline for those in need. As a dietician, my journey through the realm of nutrition had always been defined by the pursuit of knowledge, the constant quest to understand the intricate dance between food and health. But little did I know that a singular moment of revelation would lead me to pen the book you now hold in your hands: "The Low-Potassium Food List."

It was a warm summer's day, and I found myself, quite unexpectedly, in the bustling heart of a local farmers' market. Vibrant stalls, brimming with fresh produce and the heady scent of ripe fruits, drew my attention. My career, which had primarily revolved around the myriad dimensions of nutrition, had seemingly overlooked an enigma – the role of potassium in our diets.

As I wandered through the colourful aisles, my gaze was drawn to an elderly woman who was intently selecting her fruits. She was scrutinizing the labels, meticulously inspecting each item as if it held the key to her very life. Her face reflected a quiet determination, a resolve that had been etched by years of grappling with an invisible foe.

With an air of hesitant curiosity, I approached her, and our conversation unfurled like the petals of a rare and delicate flower. She introduced herself as Anne, and her eyes gleamed with a flicker of hope. Anne was in her eighties, a testament to resilience, and she harboured a deep-seated knowledge about the intricacies of a low-potassium diet that would astound me. Her life had become a delicate balancing act, a tightrope walks on which she navigated the treacherous waters of kidney disease. It was a path laden with sacrifices, of foods she had loved but could no longer Savor.

As Anne shared her story, I was struck by the staggering lack of resources and information available to her. The agony of constant trial and error, the fear of inadvertently consuming forbidden fruits – these were daily struggles she and countless others faced. I was inspired by her unwavering determination, her resolute spirit to lead a life of quality even when faced with a daunting health challenge. The challenges she confronted, the anxiety that gripped her whenever she approached her plate, all bore witness to the profound impact of potassium on our well-being.

With Anne's narrative resonating in my heart, I embarked on a journey of discovery. I delved into the intricate world of low-potassium foods, and as the layers of this enigmatic puzzle began to unravel, my mission crystallized: to compile a comprehensive and accessible resource, a beacon of hope for individuals like Anne who grapple with dietary restrictions imposed by the silent sentinel, potassium.

"The Low-Potassium Food List" is not just a book; it is a lifeline, a heartfelt offering to those who seek a better quality of life through informed choices. Within these pages, you will find an extensive catalog of low-potassium foods, delectable recipes, and a treasure trove of knowledge designed to empower you. I have poured my heart and soul into this work, and I am determined to ensure that no one faces the challenges of low potassium living alone.

Through my journey, I've discovered that knowledge is the key to liberation. We can unlock the shackles of anxiety, banish the clouds of uncertainty, and revel in the joys of a well-curated diet that supports our health. In "The Low-Potassium Food List," you will find not just a compendium of facts, but a handcrafted guide born from empathy and experience.

In the chapters that follow, you will navigate a realm of low-potassium wonders. You will Savor the Flavors of nourishing dishes, explore the depths of ingredient lists, and gain insights that will fundamentally alter the way you view your plate. Here, you will be introduced to a world where culinary pleasures harmonize seamlessly with dietary necessities.

I encourage you to embark on this transformative journey with me, for the pursuit of health is a voyage, not a destination. I am here to guide you, to be your companion on this path of knowledge and wellness. I promise you, there is no need to walk it alone.

So, whether you're a seasoned traveler through the world of low-potassium eating or a newcomer seeking answers, I welcome you to "The Low-Potassium Food List." Together, we shall redefine the boundaries of nutrition, break down the walls of dietary limitation, and chart a course toward a brighter, healthier future.

As you turn the page and begin your adventure with me, remember that knowledge is power, and together, we hold the key to a life well-lived, free from the constraints of low-potassium anxiety. Welcome to the journey of a lifetime.

CHAPTER 1

What is Potassium?

Potassium is an essential mineral and electrolyte that plays a crucial role in various physiological functions within the human body. It is indicated on the periodic table with the symbol "K" and has an atomic number of 19. Potassium is an alkali metal and is highly reactive, making it a vital component of various biological processes.

Here are some key aspects of potassium:

Function in the Body: Potassium is primarily found within cells and is involved in maintaining the body's fluid balance, nerve signaling, and muscle contractions, including the beating of the heart. It also helps regulate blood pressure and plays a role in acid-base balance.

Dietary Sources: Potassium is naturally present in a wide range of foods, with particularly high levels in fruits and vegetables such as bananas, oranges, potatoes, spinach, and avocados. Other sources include dairy products, meat, and fish.

Recommended Daily Intake: The recommended daily intake of potassium for adults is typically around 2,600-3,400 milligrams, although individual needs may vary based on factors like age, sex, and overall health.

Why is Low Potassium Important?

Low potassium levels, a condition known as hypokalemia, can have significant health implications:

Muscle Weakness: Insufficient potassium can lead to muscle weakness and cramps because potassium is essential for muscle contraction. Severe cases may even result in paralysis.

Fatigue: Low potassium levels can cause fatigue and weakness, making it challenging to perform everyday tasks and exercise.

Irregular Heartbeat: Potassium is essential for maintaining a regular heartbeat. Low levels can disrupt the heart's electrical activity, potentially leading to arrhythmias or other serious cardiac issues.

Kidney Problems: Kidneys play a crucial role in regulating potassium levels in the body. Chronic kidney disease can result in potassium buildup or loss, which can be harmful.

Digestive Issues: Low potassium can lead to digestive problems like constipation.

Increased Blood Pressure: In some cases, low potassium levels may contribute to high blood pressure.

Who Should Follow a Low Potassium Diet?

A low potassium diet is typically recommended for individuals who have hyperkalemia, a condition characterized by elevated levels of potassium in the blood. Those who may need to limit their potassium intake include:

People with Kidney Problems: Individuals with kidney disease, particularly advanced stages, may have difficulty excreting excess potassium. Therefore, they may need to restrict their dietary potassium intake to avoid hyperkalemia.

Certain Medications: Some medications, such as certain types of diuretics and medications that spare potassium, can cause potassium levels to rise. In such cases, a low potassium diet may be advised.

Potassium is a vital mineral with multiple functions in the body, and low potassium levels can have adverse effects, particularly on muscle function and heart health. While most people need an adequate intake of potassium, individuals with certain health conditions, such as kidney problems or those taking specific medications, may be advised to follow a low potassium diet to manage their potassium levels effectively.

CHAPTER 2
LOW-POTASSIUM FOOD
CATEGORIES

Low-Potassium Fruits

Strawberries:

- Potassium: 153 mg
- Calories: 32
- Carbohydrates: 7.7 g
- Fiber: 2 g
- Vitamin C: 59 mg

Blueberries:

- Potassium: 77 mg
- Calories: 57
- Carbohydrates: 14.5 g
- Fiber: 2.4 g
- Vitamin C: 9.7 mg

Raspberries:

- Potassium: 151 mg
- Calories: 52
- Carbohydrates: 11.9 g
- Fiber: 6.5 g
- Vitamin C: 26.2 mg

Blackberries:

- Potassium: 233 mg
- Calories: 43
- Carbohydrates: 9.6 g
- Fiber: 5.3 g
- Vitamin C: 21 mg

Cranberries:

- Potassium: 85 mg
- Calories: 46
- Carbohydrates: 12.2 g
- Fiber: 4.6 g
- Vitamin C: 13.3 mg

Apples:

- Potassium: 107 mg
- Calories: 52
- Carbohydrates: 14 g
- Fiber: 2.4 g
- Vitamin C: 0.5 mg

Pears:

- Potassium: 119 mg
- Calories: 57
- Carbohydrates: 15.5 g
- Fiber: 3.1 g
- Vitamin C: 4.2 mg

Kiwi:

- Potassium: 312 mg
- Calories: 61
- Carbohydrates: 14.6 g
- Fiber: 3 g
- Vitamin C: 92.7 mg

Watermelon:

- Potassium: 112 mg
- Calories: 30
- Carbohydrates: 7.6 g
- Fiber: 0.4 g
- Vitamin C: 8.1 mg

Papaya:

- Potassium: 182 mg
- Calories: 43
- Carbohydrates: 11 g
- Fiber: 1.7 g
- Vitamin C: 60.9 mg

Apricots:

- Potassium: 259 mg
- Calories: 48
- Carbohydrates: 11.1 g
- Fiber: 2 g
- Vitamin C: 10.6 mg

Peaches:

- Potassium: 190 mg
- Calories: 39
- Carbohydrates: 9.5 g
- Fiber: 1.5 g
- Vitamin C: 6.6 mg

Nectarines:

- Potassium: 201 mg
- Calories: 44
- Carbohydrates: 10.6 g
- Fiber: 1.7 g
- Vitamin C: 5.4 mg

Cherries:

- Potassium: 222 mg
- Calories: 50
- Carbohydrates: 12.2 g
- Fiber: 1.6 g
- Vitamin C: 7 mg

Mangoes:

- Potassium: 168 mg
- Calories: 60
- Carbohydrates: 14.6 g
- Fiber: 1.6 g
- Vitamin C: 36.4 mg

Low-Potassium Vegetables

Cucumber:

- Potassium: 147 mg
- Calories: 15
- Carbohydrates: 3.6 g
- Fiber: 0.5 g
- Vitamin K: 16.4 mcg

Zucchini (Courgette):

- Potassium: 261 mg
- Calories: 17
- Carbohydrates: 3.1 g
- Fiber: 1 g
- Vitamin C: 17.9 mg

Green Beans:

- Potassium: 209 mg
- Calories: 31
- Carbohydrates: 7.1 g
- Fiber: 2.7 g
- Vitamin K: 14.4 mcg

Cauliflower:

- Potassium: 299 mg
- Calories: 25
- Carbohydrates: 5.3 g
- Fiber: 2 g
- Vitamin C: 48.2 mg

Eggplant (Aubergine):

- Potassium: 229 mg
- Calories: 25
- Carbohydrates: 6 g
- Fiber: 3 g
- Vitamin C: 2.2 mg

Bell Peppers (Red, Green, Yellow):

- Potassium: 175 mg
- Calories: 31
- Carbohydrates: 6.3 g
- Fiber: 2.1 g
- Vitamin C: 128.7 mg

Spinach:

- Potassium: 558 mg
- Calories: 23
- Carbohydrates: 3.6 g
- Fiber: 2.2 g
- Vitamin A: 9377 IU

Kale:

- Potassium: 491 mg
- Calories: 49
- Carbohydrates: 8.8 g
- Fiber: 2 g
- Vitamin K: 817 mcg

Lettuce (Iceberg):

- Potassium: 141 mg
- Calories: 14
- Carbohydrates: 2.9 g
- Fiber: 1 g
- Vitamin A: 245 IU

Celery:

- Potassium: 260 mg
- Calories: 16
- Carbohydrates: 3 g
- Fiber: 1.6 g
- Vitamin K: 29.3 mcg

Asparagus:

- Potassium: 202 mg
- Calories: 20
- Carbohydrates: 3.7 g
- Fiber: 2.1 g
- Vitamin K: 41.6 mcg

Radishes:

- Potassium: 233 mg
- Calories: 16
- Carbohydrates: 3.4 g
- Fiber: 1.6 g
- Vitamin C: 14.8 mg

Carrots:

- Potassium: 320 mg
- Calories: 41
- Carbohydrates: 10 g
- Fiber: 2.8 g
- Vitamin A: 16706 IU

Broccoli:

- Potassium: 316 mg
- Calories: 55
- Carbohydrates: 11.2 g
- Fiber: 3.3 g
- Vitamin C: 89.2 mg

Onions:

- Potassium: 146 mg
- Calories: 40
- Carbohydrates: 9.3 g
- Fiber: 1.7 g
- Vitamin C: 7.4 mg

Low-Potassium Protein

Chicken Breast (skinless, boneless):

- Protein: 31 grams
- Calories: 165
- Fat: 3.6 grams
- Sodium: 74 mg

Turkey Breast (skinless, boneless):

- Protein: 29 grams
- Calories: 135
- Fat: 0.7 grams
- Sodium: 43 mg

Pork Tenderloin:

- Protein: 22 grams
- Calories: 143
- Fat: 3.6 grams
- Sodium: 48 mg

Lean Beef (Top Round or Sirloin):

- Protein: 31 grams
- Calories: 143
- Fat: 3.5 grams
- Sodium: 46 mg

Tofu (firm):

- Protein: 15 grams
- Calories: 144
- Fat: 8 grams
- Sodium: 11 mg

Tempeh:

- Protein: 19 grams
- Calories: 193
- Fat: 11 grams
- Sodium: 9 mg

Skinless Salmon:

- Protein: 25 grams
- Calories: 206
- Fat: 13 grams
- Sodium: 51 mg

Skinless Whitefish (e.g., Cod or Haddock):

- Protein: 18 grams
- Calories: 88
- Fat: 0.7 grams
- Sodium: 64 mg

Shrimp:

- Protein: 24 grams
- Calories: 99
- Fat: 1.5 grams
- Sodium: 119 mg

Eggs (boiled or poached):

- Protein: 13 grams
- Calories: 155
- Fat: 11 grams
- Sodium: 124 mg

Low-Fat Cottage Cheese:

- Protein: 12 grams
- Calories: 72
- Fat: 1 gram
- Sodium: 459 mg

Skinless Turkey Drumstick:

- Protein: 28 grams
- Calories: 135
- Fat: 2.2 grams
- Sodium: 49 mg

Skinless Chicken Thigh (boneless):

- Protein: 21 grams
- Calories: 119
- Fat: 4.3 grams
- Sodium: 50 mg

Low-Fat Greek Yogurt:

- Protein: 10 grams
- Calories: 59
- Fat: 0.4 grams
- Sodium: 41 mg

Skinless Duck Breast:

- Protein: 17 grams
- Calories: 149
- Fat: 6 grams
- Sodium: 52 mg

Low-Potassium Dairy and Alternatives

Skim Milk:

- Potassium: 132 mg
- Calories: 34
- Protein: 3.4 grams
- Fat: 0.2 grams
- Calcium: 125 mg

Low-Fat Yogurt (Plain):

- Potassium: 141 mg
- Calories: 63
- Protein: 4.5 grams
- Fat: 1.5 grams
- Calcium: 183 mg

Cottage Cheese (Low-Fat):

- Potassium: 86 mg
- Calories: 72
- Protein: 12 grams
- Fat: 1 gram
- Calcium: 76 mg

Mozzarella Cheese (Part-Skim):

- Potassium: 156 mg
- Calories: 254
- Protein: 24 grams
- Fat: 15 grams
- Calcium: 731 mg

Ricotta Cheese (Part-Skim):

- Potassium: 138 mg
- Calories: 138
- Protein: 14 grams
- Fat: 8 grams
- Calcium: 337 mg

Almond Milk (Unsweetened):

- Potassium: 180 mg
- Calories: 13
- Protein: 0.5 grams
- Fat: 1.2 grams
- Calcium: 516 mg

Soy Milk (Unsweetened):

- Potassium: 117 mg
- Calories: 33
- Protein: 3.3 grams
- Fat: 1.4 grams
- Calcium: 299 mg

Rice Milk (Unsweetened):

- Potassium: 47 mg
- Calories: 47
- Protein: 0.3 grams
- Fat: 1 gram
- Calcium: 283 mg

Oat Milk (Unsweetened):

- Potassium: 74 mg
- Calories: 40
- Protein: 1 gram
- Fat: 1.5 grams
- Calcium: 370 mg

Coconut Milk (Canned, Unsweetened):

- Potassium: 170 mg
- Calories: 230
- Protein: 2.3 grams
- Fat: 23 grams
- Calcium: 15 mg

Hemp Milk (Unsweetened):

- Potassium: 51 mg
- Calories: 49
- Protein: 2 grams
- Fat: 4 grams
- Calcium: 300 mg

Cashew Milk (Unsweetened):

- Potassium: 30 mg
- Calories: 25
- Protein: 0 grams
- Fat: 2 grams
- Calcium: 30 mg

Greek Yogurt (Dairy-Free, Plant-Based):

- Potassium: Varies by brand
- Calories: Varies by brand
- Protein: Varies by brand
- Fat: Varies by brand
- Calcium: Varies by brand

Coconut Yogurt (Dairy-Free, Plant-Based):

- Potassium: Varies by brand
- Calories: Varies by brand
- Protein: Varies by brand
- Fat: Varies by brand
- Calcium: Varies by brand

Almond-based Cheese (Dairy-Free):

- Potassium: Varies by brand
- Calories: Varies by brand
- Protein: Varies by brand
- Fat: Varies by brand
- Calcium: Varies by brand

Low-Potassium Grains and Cereals

White Rice (cooked):

- Potassium: 43 mg
- Calories: 130
- Carbohydrates: 28.7 grams
- Fiber: 0.4 grams
- Protein: 2.7 grams

Pasta (cooked):

- Potassium: 25 mg
- Calories: 131
- Carbohydrates: 25.0 grams
- Fiber: 1.3 grams
- Protein: 4.5 grams

Oatmeal (cooked):

- Potassium: 71 mg
- Calories: 71
- Carbohydrates: 12.4 grams
- Fiber: 1.7 grams
- Protein: 2.5 grams

Barley (cooked):

- Potassium: 93 mg
- Calories: 96
- Carbohydrates: 21.7 grams
- Fiber: 3 grams
- Protein: 2.3 grams

Quinoa (cooked):

- Potassium: 172 mg
- Calories: 120
- Carbohydrates: 21.3 grams
- Fiber: 2.8 grams
- Protein: 4.1 grams

Farro (cooked):

- Potassium: 141 mg
- Calories: 170
- Carbohydrates: 35.7 grams
- Fiber: 4.7 grams
- Protein: 5.4 grams

Couscous (cooked):

- Potassium: 6 mg
- Calories: 176
- Carbohydrates: 36.5 grams
- Fiber: 2.2 grams
- Protein: 6 grams

Bulgur (cooked):

- Potassium: 20 mg
- Calories: 83
- Carbohydrates: 18.6 grams
- Fiber: 4.1 grams
- Protein: 3.1 grams

Cornmeal (cooked):

- Potassium: 109 mg
- Calories: 123
- Carbohydrates: 25.2 grams
- Fiber: 1.6 grams
- Protein: 3.2 grams

Millet (cooked):

- Potassium: 119 mg
- Calories: 119
- Carbohydrates: 25.7 grams
- Fiber: 1.3 grams
- Protein: 3.5 grams

White Bread:

- Potassium: 108 mg
- Calories: 265
- Carbohydrates: 49.4 grams
- Fiber: 2.4 grams
- Protein: 8.3 grams

Rye Bread:

- Potassium: 125 mg
- Calories: 259
- Carbohydrates: 51.2 grams
- Fiber: 6.1 grams
- Protein: 7.8 grams

Corn Flakes Cereal:

- Potassium: 63 mg
- Calories: 365
- Carbohydrates: 84.0 grams
- Fiber: 1.3 grams
- Protein: 6.6 grams

Rice Cakes:

- Potassium: 33 mg
- Calories: 35
- Carbohydrates: 7.3 grams
- Fiber: 0.2 grams
- Protein: 0.8 grams

Plain Popcorn (air-popped):

Potassium: 153 mg

Calories: 387

Carbohydrates: 78.1 grams

Fiber: 15.1 grams

Protein: 12.9 grams

Low-Potassium Snacks and Sweets

Pretzels:

- Potassium: 68 mg
- Calories: 384
- Carbohydrates: 80.5 grams
- Fat: 1.3 grams
- Protein: 9.1 grams

Rice Cakes:

- Potassium: 24 mg
- Calories: 387
- Carbohydrates: 82.0 grams
- Fat: 2.1 grams
- Protein: 7.5 grams

Plain Popcorn (air-popped):

- Potassium: 153 mg
- Calories: 387
- Carbohydrates: 78.1 grams
- Fat: 4.3 grams
- Protein: 12.9 grams

Graham Crackers:

- Potassium: 94 mg
- Calories: 386
- Carbohydrates: 78.8 grams
- Fat: 8.6 grams
- Protein: 4.7 grams

Rice Krispies Treats:

- Potassium: 60 mg
- Calories: 402
- Carbohydrates: 84.3 grams
- Fat: 6.7 grams
- Protein: 2.6 grams

Jellybeans:

- Potassium: 1 mg
- Calories: 375
- Carbohydrates: 94.2 grams
- Fat: 0.5 grams
- Protein: 0.9 grams

Hard Candy (Assorted):

- Potassium: 2 mg
- Calories: 394
- Carbohydrates: 97.3 grams
- Fat: 0 grams
- Protein: 0 grams

Marshmallows:

- Potassium: 54 mg
- Calories: 318
- Carbohydrates: 81.4 grams
- Fat: 0.1 grams
- Protein: 0.8 grams

Gummy Bears:

- Potassium: 36 mg
- Calories: 325
- Carbohydrates: 80.5 grams
- Fat: 0.2 grams
- Protein: 2.5 grams

Licorice (Twizzlers):

- Potassium: 10 mg
- Calories: 349
- Carbohydrates: 86.9 grams
- Fat: 0.9 grams
- Protein: 1.2 grams

Fruit Flavored Gelatin (Sugar-Free):

- Potassium: 53 mg
- Calories: 5
- Carbohydrates: 0.4 grams
- Fat: 0 grams
- Protein: 1 gram

Angel Food Cake:

- Potassium: 123 mg
- Calories: 206
- Carbohydrates: 47.6 grams
- Fat: 0.6 grams
- Protein: 4.4 grams

Shortbread Cookies:

- Potassium: 88 mg
- Calories: 501
- Carbohydrates: 63.5 grams
- Fat: 25.6 grams
- Protein: 5.9 grams

Fruit Sorbet (Various Flavors):

- Potassium: Varies by flavor
- Calories: Varies by flavor
- Carbohydrates: Varies by flavor
- Fat: Varies by flavor
- Protein: Varies by flavor

Vanilla Pudding (Sugar-Free):

- Potassium: 73 mg
- Calories: 88
- Carbohydrates: 7.8 grams
- Fat: 3.4 grams
- Protein: 5.2 grams

CONCLUSION

In the realm of low potassium living, we have journeyed together through pages filled with knowledge, compassion, and hope. As we reach the conclusion of our voyage, I am humbled by the profound connection we have established.

"The Low-Potassium Food List" is more than just a book; it is a testament to the strength of the human spirit, the enduring will to transcend adversity, and the boundless capacity for growth and transformation. It is a declaration that knowledge is a beacon of light, illuminating the darkest corners of our health challenges.

Throughout this book, we have uncovered the secrets of low potassium living, learned to navigate the dietary landscape, and celebrated the beauty of culinary creativity within these constraints. We have shared stories, tasted the flavors of nourishing dishes, and felt the warmth of a community that stands together in the face of challenges.

As we part ways, I urge you to remember that the journey does not end here. It is an ongoing exploration, a continuous evolution of understanding, and a commitment to nurturing your well-being. You are not alone on this path, for the knowledge you have gained and the choices you make have the power to transform not just your life, but the lives of those around you.

The low-potassium journey can be challenging, but it is a journey of strength, resilience, and discovery. It is an exploration of the profound connection between what we eat and how we live. It is a reminder that every meal we choose is a step toward health and vitality.

In closing, I want you to carry with you the understanding that you hold the power to create your own narrative of health, to craft your own story of well-being. The pages of this book are but a prologue to the boundless possibilities that await you. Embrace your newfound knowledge, savor the flavors of your meals, and relish in the simplicity and beauty of living well.

Thank you for allowing me to be a part of your journey, for sharing in the joys and challenges of low potassium living, and for taking the steps to transform your health and enhance the quality of your life. May your path be one of vitality, and may your future be filled with the brightest of tomorrows.

Farewell, dear reader, and may your heart be forever nourished, your spirit forever uplifted, and your life forever enriched by the journey we have taken together.

BONUS:

10 LOW-POTASSIUM RECIPES

Grilled Chicken Breast with Lemon and Herbs

Cooking Time: 20 minutes

Servings: 4

Ingredients:

- 4 boneless, skinless chicken breasts (4 oz each)
- 1 lemon, juiced.
- 2 cloves garlic, minced.
- 2 tablespoons fresh herbs (e.g., rosemary, thyme, or oregano)
- 1 tablespoon olive oil
- Salt and pepper to taste

Instructions:

1. Preheat the grill to medium-high heat.
2. In a bowl, mix the lemon juice, minced garlic, fresh herbs, and olive oil.
3. Season the chicken breasts with salt and pepper, then brush them with the lemon herb mixture.

4. Grill the chicken for about 5-7 minutes on each side or until fully cooked.

5. Serve with a side of steamed green beans and brown rice.

Nutritional Information (per serving):

Calories: 190

Protein: 26 grams

Carbohydrates: 2 grams

Fat: 9 grams

Fiber: 1 gram

Potassium: Approximately 170 mg

Baked Salmon with Dill

Cooking Time: 25 minutes

Servings: 4

Ingredients:

- 4 salmon fillets (4 oz each)
- 2 tablespoons fresh dill, chopped.
- 1 lemon, sliced.
- Salt and pepper to taste

Instructions:

1. Preheat the oven to 375°F (190°C).
2. Season the salmon fillets with salt, pepper, and chopped dill.
3. Place a slice of lemon on each fillet.
4. Wrap the salmon in foil and bake for about 20 minutes or until the salmon flakes easily.
5. Serve with a side of quinoa and steamed asparagus.

Nutritional Information (per serving):

Calories: 180

Protein: 24 grams

Carbohydrates: 6 grams

Fat: 7 grams

Fiber: 2 grams

Potassium: Approximately 260 mg

Quinoa and Black Bean Salad

Cooking Time: 20 minutes

Servings: 4

Ingredients:

- 1 cup quinoa cooked and cooled.
- 1 can (15 oz) low-sodium black beans, drained and rinsed.
- 1 cup cherry tomatoes, halved.
- 1/2 red onion finely chopped.
- 1/4 cup fresh cilantro, chopped.
- Juice of 2 limes
- 2 tablespoons olive oil
- Salt and pepper to taste

Instructions:

1. In a large bowl, combine quinoa, black beans, cherry tomatoes, red onion, and cilantro.
2. In a separate bowl, whisk together lime juice, olive oil, salt, and pepper.
3. Pour the dressing over the salad and toss to combine.
4. Refrigerate for at least 1 hour before serving.

Nutritional Information (per serving):

Calories: 250

Protein: 9 grams

Carbohydrates: 38 grams

Fat: 7 grams

Fiber: 7 grams

Potassium: Approximately 320 mg

Vegetable Stir-Fry

Cooking Time: 20 minutes

Servings: 4

Ingredients:

- 2 cups broccoli florets
- 1 red bell pepper, sliced.
- 1 yellow bell pepper, sliced.
- 1 zucchini, sliced.
- 1 carrot, julienned
- 1 cup snap peas
- 1 tablespoon low-sodium soy sauce
- 1 tablespoon olive oil
- 1 teaspoon ginger, minced.
- 1 clove garlic, minced.
- Salt and pepper to taste

Instructions:

1. Heat olive oil in a large skillet over medium-high heat.
2. Add ginger and garlic and sauté for about 1 minute.
3. Add all the vegetables and stir-fry for 7-10 minutes or until they are tender.

4. Drizzle with soy sauce, salt, and pepper, and cook for an additional 2 minutes.

5. Serve over brown rice or whole wheat noodles.

Nutritional Information (per serving):

Calories: 130

Protein: 4 grams

Carbohydrates: 20 grams

Fat: 5 grams

Fiber: 5 grams

Potassium: Approximately 320 mg

Turkey and Vegetable Soup

Cooking Time: 30 minutes

Servings: 6

Ingredients:

- 1 lb ground turkey
- 1 onion, chopped.
- 2 carrots, chopped.
- 2 celery stalks, chopped.
- 1 zucchini, diced.
- 1 can (15 oz) low sodium diced tomatoes.
- 6 cups low-sodium chicken broth
- 1 cup green beans, chopped.
- 1 teaspoon dried thyme
- Salt and pepper to taste

Instructions:

1. In a large pot, cook ground turkey until browned.
2. Add chopped onion, carrots, and celery, and cook until vegetables are tender.
3. Stir in zucchini, diced tomatoes, chicken broth, green beans, thyme, salt, and pepper.
4. Bring to a boil, then reduce heat and simmer for 20 minutes.
5. Serve hot.

Nutritional Information (per serving):

Calories: 210

Protein: 21 grams

Carbohydrates: 11 grams

Fat: 8 grams

Fiber: 3 grams

Potassium: Approximately 380 mg

Egg White Omelets with Spinach and Tomatoes

Cooking Time: 15 minutes

Servings: 2

Ingredients:

- 4 large egg whites
- 1 cup fresh spinach, chopped.
- 1 medium tomato, diced.
- 1/4 cup low-fat feta cheese
- Salt and pepper to taste

Instructions:

1. Whisk the egg whites in a bowl and season with salt and pepper.
2. Heat a non-stick skillet over medium heat and add the chopped spinach and tomatoes.
3. Cook for 2-3 minutes until the spinach wilts.
4. Pour the egg whites over the vegetables and cook until set.
5. Sprinkle with feta cheese and fold the omelet in half before serving.

Nutritional Information (per serving):

Calories: 120

Protein: 16 grams

Carbohydrates: 5 grams

Fat: 4 grams

Fiber: 2 grams

Potassium: Approximately 280 mg

Low-Potassium Fruit Salad

Preparation Time: 15 minutes

Servings: 4

Ingredients:

- 2 cups fresh strawberries, sliced.
- 2 cups fresh pineapple, diced.
- 2 cups fresh blueberries
- 1 cup fresh raspberries
- 1 tablespoon honey (optional)
- Fresh mint leaves for garnish

Instructions:

1. In a large bowl, combine the sliced strawberries, diced pineapple, blueberries, and raspberries.
2. Drizzle honey over the fruit if desired and gently toss to combine.
3. Garnish with fresh mint leaves.
4. Serve immediately or refrigerate for a cool and refreshing treat.

Nutritional Information (per serving):

Calories: 90

Protein: 1 gram

Carbohydrates: 22 grams

Fat: 0.5 grams

Fiber: 5 grams

Potassium: Approximately 150 mg

Low-Potassium Avocado and Tomato Salsa

Preparation Time: 15 minutes

Servings: 4

Ingredients:

- 2 ripe avocados, diced.
- 2 large tomatoes, diced.
- 1/2 red onion finely chopped.
- 1/4 cup fresh cilantro, chopped.
- Juice of 2 limes
- Salt and pepper to taste

Instructions:

1. In a bowl, gently combine the diced avocados, tomatoes, red onion, and cilantro.
2. Squeeze lime juice over the mixture, and season with salt and pepper.
3. Stir to combine and serve as a dip with whole-grain tortilla chips or as a topping for grilled chicken or fish.

Nutritional Information (per serving):

Calories: 150

Protein: 2 grams

Carbohydrates: 12 grams

Fat: 12 grams

Fiber: 7 grams

Potassium: Approximately 350 mg

Low-Potassium Tuna Salad

Preparation Time: 20 minutes

Servings: 2

Ingredients:

- 2 cans (5 oz each) low-sodium tuna, drained
- 1/2 cup cucumber, diced.
- 1/2 cup red bell pepper, diced.
- 1/4 cup red onion finely chopped.
- 2 tablespoons fresh dill, chopped.
- 1/4 cup low-fat mayonnaise
- Juice of 1 lemon
- Salt and pepper to taste

Instructions:

1. In a bowl, combine the drained tuna, diced cucumber, red bell pepper, red onion, and fresh dill.
2. Add the low-fat mayonnaise and lemon juice and mix until well combined.
3. Season with salt and pepper to taste.
4. Serve as a sandwich filling or on a bed of fresh lettuce.

Nutritional Information (per serving):

Calories: 260

Protein: 23 grams

Carbohydrates: 8 grams

Fat: 15 grams

Fiber: 2 grams

Potassium: Approximately 300 mg

Low-Potassium Baked Sweet Potatoes

Preparation Time: 45 minutes

Servings: 4

Ingredients:

- 4 small sweet potatoes
- 1 tablespoon olive oil
- Salt and pepper to taste
- Fresh rosemary sprigs (optional)

Instructions:

1. Preheat the oven to 400°F (200°C).
2. Scrub the sweet potatoes and pierce them with a fork several times.
3. Rub each sweet potato with a bit of olive oil, and season with salt and pepper.
4. Place the sweet potatoes on a baking sheet and bake for about 40-45 minutes or until they are soft and easily pierced with a fork.
5. Garnish with fresh rosemary sprigs if desired.

Nutritional Information (per serving):

Calories: 100

Protein: 1 gram

Carbohydrates: 23 grams

Fat: 1 gram

Fiber: 4 grams

Potassium: Approximately 180 mg

Printed in Great Britain
by Amazon

46745795R00040